AF659384

Instructional Modules For AIDS Education

INTERNATIONAL ENCYCLOPAEDIA OF AIDS-10

INSTRUCTIONAL MODULES FOR AIDS EDUCATION

Editor
Dr. Digumarti Bhaskara Rao
M.Sc. , M.A., M.A., M.Ed., Ph.D.
R. V. R. College of Education
Guntur–522 006
Andhra Pradesh. (INDIA)

2000
DISCOVERY PUBLISHING HOUSE
NEW DELHI-110 002

First Published-2000

ISBN 81-7141-532-6

© Editor

Published by:
DISCOVERY PUBLISHING HOUSE
48[illegible]1/24, Ansari Road, Prahlad Street,
Darya Ganj, New Delhi-110 002 (*INDIA*)
Phone: 3279245
Fax: 91-11-3253475

Printed at:
Arora Offset Press
Laxmi Nagar, Delhi 110 092.

PREFACE

The HIV/AIDS is a new phenomenon in the human society. HIV destroys the immune system of human individuals, producing a defenselessness fatal state known as AIDS. The World Health Organisation has estimated that already one in every two hundred and fifty adults in the world is infected with Human Immunodeficiency Virus and according to WHO's projections a total of forty million men women and children worldwide will have been infected with HIV by the turn of this twentieth century. Visualising the devastating effects of the HIV/AIDS epidemic within our life times and beyond is difficult. Probably, no other disease in recent times has had the impact on human society generated by HIV/AIDS.

The HIV/AIDS epidemic has brought into focus many health related ethical, legal and human rights issues. This epidemic requires immediate and effective responses in new programming areas: attitudinal and behavioural changes, community-based care and support initiatives, and the maintenance of human development in the face of increasing rates of illness and deaths. At this point, education enters the scene as it can alter the HIV/AIDS situation since it brings change in the behaviour of the people.

This *International Encyclopaedia of AIDS* presents the worldwide information about HIV/AIDS, issues and challenges, reports and reviews, ethics laws and human rights, and educational activities and programmes to keep the policy makers, planners, professionals, activists, researchers, educationists, teachers and students well informed of the epidemic.

Dr. Digumarti Bhaskara Rao
26 January 1999
The Republic Day of India

ACKNOWLEDGEMENT

I am thankful to the World Health Organisation and its associated offices for using their material namely School Health Education to prevent AIDS and STD: A Resource Package for Curriculum Planners-Handbook for Curriculum Planners. Student's Activities, Teachers' Guide, Global Programme on AIDS-HIV Prevention and Care: Teaching Modules for Nurses and Midwives, Global Programme on AIDS. Community HIV Prevention Handbook; STD care Management-workbooks 1-7, Facing the Challenge of HIV/ AIDS STDs: A Gender-based Response; HIV/AIDS and STD surveillance Data Management and Use-Report, Bangkok, 1995; Carrying out HIV Sentinal Surveillance-A Guide for Programme Managers, AIDS Prevention and Care in the workplace: Enhancing the Role of Private Sector; HIV Testing Policies and Guidelines; Carrying out HIV Sentinel surveillance; AIDS Prevention; Understanding and Living with AIDS; AIDS: A Modern Epidemic; HIV/AIDS in South-East Asia: IXth meeting of the National Programme Managers, New Delhi, 1993; Information, Education and Communication: A Guide for AIDS Programme Managers, Handbook on AIDS Home Care; HIV/AIDS in South-East Asia: A Pictorial summary; etc.

I am thankful to the United Nations Development Programme, UNDP's HIV and Development Programme, and UNDP's Regional Projects on HIV and Development for using their material namely Economic Implications of AIDS in Asia; Socio Economic Implications of the Epidemic; NGOs Working with Sex workers; NGO Responses to HIV/AIDS in Asia-Case Studies; HIV in the Workplace: Dealing with the Issues-Role Plays, Development and the HIV Epidemic, Law Ethics and HIV; HIV Law and Law Reform; Issue Papers; Study Papers; Working Papers; etc.

I am thankful to the Health and Nutrition Centre, Republic of Philippines for using its material namely sourcebook on HIV/AIDS Prevention Education for Tertiary Educational Institutions.

I am thankful to the Curriculum Development Programme, Ministry of Education, Government of Thailand for using its material namely Institutional Modules for AIDS Education.

I am thankful to US Department of Health and Human Services: Whitman-Walker Clinic, Inc., USA; East-West Centre, USA; National AIDS Control Organisation, Government of India; Academy of Culture Communication Education Science and Service, Guntur, United Nations and its agencies for using their material.

I am grateful to Bhaskar Bhattacharji; V. Alexeev, Geeta Sethi, Elizabeth Reid, Mina Mauerstein-Bail, A. A. Trinidad, Palomi Cuchi, D. Pushpa Latha for their kind co-operation.

Dr. Digumarti Bhaskara Rao,
Secretary
ACCESS
D-43, S.V. N. Colony,
Guntur-522 006

CONTENTS

1

INTRODUCTION

MODULE SECTIONS

Each module is comprised of the following main sections:

1. *Topic*: Each topic is named to ensure consistency of content as well as to stimulate both teachers and students.

2. *Content*: It is important for the teacher to have a thorough understanding of the concepts introduced in each instructional module and to consider the means to summarize them.

3. *Objectives*: These are expressed as types of student behaviour that indicate whether, after doing the recommended activities, they have achieved the set objectives.

4. *Teaching activities*: The activities are presented in sequence, and comprise three steps:

   a) The initial step, *Stimulating and Creating Interest*, can be accomplished through establishing an atmosphere and environment that foster learning, such as arranging student desks in a certain way, putting up some pictures, using leading questions, and talking about news and current events.

b) The activity step, *Instructional Presentation*, comprises various types of teaching and learning activities, including

- Case study
- Role play
- Simulation
- Play
- Group discussion
- Research
- Games
- Group interaction

c) The Conclusion and Application step comes after students have completed all the activities. They should be able to do this on their own, but the teacher may assist if necessary. In this step, students are encouraged to apply what they have learned to their personal benefit.

5. *Teaching materials*: In each instructional module, materials and readings that relate to recommended activities are suggested, and may be adapted by the teacher as appropriate. The sources of information are included at the end of this book.

6. *Evaluation*: Emphasis is placed on cbservation of students and their work and self-evaluation.

7. *Additional suggested activities*: This section is aimed at improving the effectiveness of teaching and learning, and fostering cooperation among students, teachers, school administrators, and the community in the prevention of AIDS.

8. *Addendum*: The addendum includes worksheets and various forms that appear at the end of each teaching unit, which the teacher should prepare prior to teaching the unit.

Time Required

Three periods are required for each module, totalling 60 periods for the 20 modules. The topics are listed below:

1. What is AIDS?
2. Let's Unite in Our Efforts to Fight AIDS
3. Love Your Life, Fight AIDS
4. Love Your Life, Don't Even Consider Getting AIDS
5. If There's Life; There's Hope
6. Have Empathy Towards Others
7. Knowing Our Bodies
8. A Closely-Knit Family Can Easily Fight AIDS
9. Nit-noi Goes to the Doctor
10. Meet in the Middle
11. We Don't Want to Contract AIDS
12. AIDS is Preventable
13. AIDS is a Danger to Life and Society
14. Protect Yourself from AIDS
15. Leading a Good Life that is Free from AIDS
16. Happy Family, Free from AIDS
17. Healthy Practices Can Prevent AIDS
18. Reason and its Application will Save You from AIDS
19. Self-Control can Prevent One from Contracting AIDS
20. Leading an Ethical Life Helps Prevent AIDS

ARRANGING THE TEACHING SCHEDULE

Whether the instructional modules are included in relevant units or are taught separately, the teacher may organize the time as follows:

1. Teach the ten modules one after the other until completed, which requires two weeks.

2. Devote one hour a week until the ten topics are covered. This will take 10 weeks.

3. Devote a few hours each week on the topics until completed.

4. During the period in which the Department of Instructional Development is trying out the modules, the teacher may carry out the teaching in a manner that best suits the school situation,

OBJECTIVES OF THESE MODULES

To develop in the students:

1. Knowledge and understanding about AIDS

2. Values and attitudes towards appropriate conduct to ensure a good quality of life for one's self, one's family, and the society

3. A healthy lifestyle

4. Self-control, awareness and wisdom to solve problems in the face of temptation.

Note: The next 20 Chapters explain the 20 modules of this programme.

2

WHAT IS AIDS?

Content:

AIDS is a fatal disease that is incurable but preventable.

Objectives:

To be able to:

- give a definition of AIDS;
- specify the cause of AIDS;
- describe the symptoms of AIDS;
- analyze and summarize news about AIDS.

Teaching activities:

1. Distribute "Mo's Story" for the students to read. Ask a student to read it aloud to the class.

2. Lead a discussion about the story, using questions to assess the students' attitudes and knowledge about AIDS at the same time.

Question: How to you feel about Mo's story?

Answer: The answers may be positive, such as a feeling of being sympathetic, which is desirable. But if the answers are negative, such as a feeling that Mo deserves his fate, the teacher then has to work towards changing the students' attitudes. The students may be asked to put themselves in Mo's place or that of Mo's family's so that they can express themselves more acceptably. They might say that it is a matter of karma. The teacher then can explain that everything has a cause. In Mo's case, it should be clear to the students that Mo contracted AIDS from her mother.

Question: Why did the French couple return Mo to Thailand?

Answer: Because the blood test results revealed that Mo was HIV positive.

Question: Do you know what being HIV positive means?

Answer: There are two steps in blood testing. The initial step, which is very simple, is to check for HIV antibodies in the blood. It takes from 24 to 48 hours to determine the result of this test. If the test result is positive, another test has to be done to confirm it. The second test is much more complex and costly, and it takes about 3-4 weeks to determine the result. If this test is positive, then it is confirmed that the person is infected with HIV, transmitted through blood contact or sexual relations or at birth from the mother.

3. Distribute the comic strip "AIDS THREAT" to read, after which students are asked what information they obtained. The answers may include the meaning of AIDS, its spread and its prevention. In addition, ask these questions:

Question: Have you ever heard these terms before? Do you know their meanings?

- Birth control - Blood test after marriage

- AIDS infection - Blood positive for HIV

Answer: Students may have heard the terms but do not know thei r meanings .

Question: Are these terms related to AIDS? How?

4. Divide the students into four groups. Distribute information sheets about AIDS to study and prepare a report for the next class.

   Group 1: The AIDS situation

   Group 2: The meaning of AIDS

   Group 3: AIDS transmission

   Group 4: AIDS symptoms

Teaching materials:

1. Case study: "Mo's Story"
2. Comic strip: "AIDS Threat"
3. AIDS pamphlets and information sheets

Evaluation:

1. Observe students' participation in class activities
2. Check students' answers from the AIDS test

Suggestions for additional activities:

1. Bulletin board arrangement
2. Gather AIDS news and organize the clippings into a book or scrapbook

ACTIVITIES

MO'S STORY

I don't know how I was born. I was saved from a garbage pile by an old lady who was very poor and could hardly take care of herself. She took me to the police, after which I was sent to an orphanage in Chiang Mai.

Why couldn't my parents take care of me? If they didn't want me, why didn't they practice birth control? Maybe they wanted to have me, but after I was born I was sickly, so they decided to discard me. Before they had me, I wonder whether they ever had their blood checked. However, it doesn't matter now. It's no use talking about what had already happened.

A French couple came to visit our orphanage and we met. They wanted to adopt me if I did not have AIDS. The result of the blood test was negative so they took me to France with them. What good luck for Mo!

When I was nine months old, I had a blood test that was positive for HIV. I was sent for treatment at Bamrasnaradoon Hospital in Nonthaburi.

The doctor told my French parents that a baby can be born with HIV because it can be transmitted from its mother if she is infected, but that there was a 60-70 percent chance that the baby would not develop AIDS. I will have to wait until I am eighteen months old to have another blood test to know for sure whether I have AIDS. My French parents are still hopeful that I will not develop AIDS. They continue to send me money. The tour guide who took my French parents to Chiang Mai frequently comes to take me to his house. His family loves me and plays with me. I enjoy the visit. The tour guide told me that my parents would come to see me. I am not sure whether I can return to France. If I develop AIDS,I will not live long, but the faster I die, the better, so I won't suffer. If I am born again, I would like to be born from parents who know that AIDS can be passed on to the foetus and that they can prevent it.

Source: *Tasanee Sa-ngaunsat, Curriculum Development Journal, Department of Instructional Development.*

TEST

Put a √ in front of a correct statement and an × in front of a statement that is incorrect.

_______________ 1. AIDS is caused by a kind of virus.

_______________ 2. Children will not come down with AIDS.

_______________ 3. If a person is healthy, he will not become infected with AIDS.

_______________ 4. If a person is infected with HIV, he will immediately show symptoms.

_______________ 5. AIDS means having an immune system deficiency.

_______________ 6. The numberof people with AIDS in Thailand is increasing everyday.

DEFINITION OF AIDS

AIDS is the acronym for Acquired Immune Deficiency Syndrome.

A = Acquired: The condition occurs after birth and is not passed on genetically.

I = Immune: The body's immune system

D = Deficiency: A lack, degeneration, decline

S = Syndrome: Group of symptoms

AIDS means having a group of symptoms acquired from a deficiency in the body's immune system.

Causes of AIDS

1. *Medical cause*: AIDS is caused by a virus known as HIV. Once this virus enters the human body, it will destroy cells

that protect the body and attack the immune system. The body weakens and becomes easily infected by other infectious diseases.

2. *Social cause*: Infection is caused by sexual contact and also by injecting drugs into the veins, for example by drug addicts who inject heroin into their veins.

AIDS symptoms

There are three phases:

1. *Being HIV Positive*: There are no symptoms. Only blood tests for HIV can tell whether a person is infected. However, a person with HIV can transmit it to other people. He can live a healthy life without showing any symptom for about 5-8 years.

2. *Showing symptoms*: There will be symptoms, called ARC, or near AIDS, which can last 3-5 years before the next phase.

3. *Full-blown AIDS*: The person will develop many kinds of infectious diseases and cancer, and will eventually die.

3

LET'S UNITE IN OUR EFFORTS TO FIGHT AIDS

Content:

AIDS is a fatal infectious disease that is incurable but preventable.

Objectives:

To be able to:

- *describe the AIDS symptoms;*

- *differentiate between a person who is HIV Positive and someone with AIDS;*

- *explain how to prevent AIDS.*

Teaching activities:

1. Have each group representative report on the previously assigned topics:

- AIDS situation

- The definition of AIDS
- The cause of AIDS
- AIDS symptoms

Have the students ask questions at each presentation. Add more information to the students' presentation as appropriate.

Reading Passage: The AIDS Situation

> AIDS is a serious disease that threatens the life and psychological well-being of people all over the world. The number of people infected with HIV and with AIDS continues to increase. There is no cure and no vaccine to prevent AIDS. The spread of AIDS is not limited to prostitutes and drug users. People who are infected include the general population, both men and women, especially those who are sexually promiscuous. A number of housewives contract AIDS from their husbands. AIDS can also be passed on by a mother to her child. Consequently, AIDS is every family's problem.

2. Ask for volunteers, two boys and two girls, to play the game, "Trial and Error"

3. Have the students study word cards to see whether they are placed under the right topics. Ask them to explain.

4. Divde the Students into 5 groups. Have them study the passage and write down the answers to the questons.

   4.1 Symptoms of HIV intecton
   4.2 Symptoms of AIDS
   4.3 AIDS transmission
   4.4 AIDS prevention

Have a representafive from each group report to the class.

5. Have two volunteers role-play: one person with HIV and one with AIDS to show the diferences between them. Have the first student act as it she had a cold. The other should act normally. The class will say that the first student has a cold and the other is normal.

Have the same two students in front of the class one with a sign. "HIV Positive", and the other with a sign, "No HIV". Ask the students to tell the differences between them. After that, remove the signs from both students and ask the students again. The answer should be that there is no difference between them.

Help the students draw the conclusion that we usually cannot differentiate a person with HIV from the rest of the population until that person develops full-blown AIDS. People who are HIV-positive can lead normal lives for 5-8 years if they take good care of themselves. However, tbey can spread the disease. This has become a serious problem that we all have to work together to eliminate.

Teaching materials:

1. Game: "Trial and Error"
2. Prepared reading materials on AIDS
3. Wall hanging board

Evaluation:

1. Observe the students' participation and discussion and their answering of questions.

2. Check reports.

ACTIVITIES

GAME: TRIAL AND ERROR

Materials:

1. Whistles

2. Cards of words and phrases concerning the causes of AIDS, symptoms, transmission, and prevention.

Examples of word cards:

Word Cards: 4 Words

cause	symptoms	transmission	prevention

Phrase Cards: 20 Phrases

weak HIV | weight loss | fever | enlarged lymph nodes

diarrhea | rash | fungus | skin cancer | blood transfusion

have sexual intercourse with HIV-Positive or AIDS-infected person

secondary infection in lungs, brain

infected mother to her foetus

cut area exposed to AIDS-infected body fluid

share infected needle with HIV positive person

share sharp objects with infected person

no sexual promiscuity

use condom

do not share needles

do not share sharp objects

How to play the game:

1. Ask for volunteers - two boys and two girls.
2. Put up the first set of words on the board or the wall board.
3. Explain to the students how to play the game:

   3.1 Mix up the second set of words and divide them into 4-5 word sets.

   3.2 Have the students pick up a card from each set and place them under the right category until finished.

   3.3 The teacher does the timing, which is one minute from beginning to end.

ACTIVITIES

REPORT FORM

TOPIC

Group ---------------------------------- Class -----------------------------

Member 1. ---------------------------
2. ---------------------------
3. ---------------------------
4. ---------------------------
5. ---------------------------
6. ---------------------------

Summary:

1. Symptoms of a person who is HIV-Positive

----

2. Symptoms of a person with AIDS

----

3. AIDS transmission

----

4. AIDS prevention

4

LOVE YOUR LIFE, FIGHT AIDS

Content:

The spread of AIDS has a great impact upon the economy, society, family and community.

Objectives:

To be able to:

- *identify the threat of AIDS to one's health;*
- *identify the impact of AIDS upon one's family and community;*
- *express concern about the impact of AIDS upon one's self, family, and society;*
- *develop a sense of responsibility in the prevention of AIDS.*

Teaching activities:

1. Show news clippings, pictures, and situations related to AIDS.

2. Conduct a group discussion on the following topics:

Question: What is the pattern of the spread of AIDS?

Answer: There is an increase in the number of people with AIDS in all age groups.

Question: Which groups of people have more chances of spreading AIDS?

Answer: Prostitutes, both men and women, drug abusers.

Question: Who do you think has a chance of contracting AIDS?

Answer: Teachers, prostitutes, teenagers, etc. (everybody).

Question: Do you think you have a chance of becoming infected with AIDS? Why?

Answer: Yes, because..............................

No, because I am still young, etc.

Question: Do you think everybody has a chance of being infected with AIDS? Why? Give examples of risky behaviour and safe behaviour.

Answer: We all can be infected by AIDS if we do not try to avoid it. Give examples.

Question: Is it necessary for you to learn about AIDS?

Answer: Yes, so that we can learn how to protect ourselves.

3. Divide the students into 4 groups. Distribute information sheets for each group to study.

   Group 1: Danger and impact of AIDS on human life

   Group 2: Danger and impact of AIDS on the family

   Group 3: Danger and impact of AIDS on the society

Group 4: Danger and impact of AIDS on the economy

4. Help the students reach the conclusion that AIDS is dangerous. Point out the impact on individuals, family, society, and the economy. (Emphasize shared responsibility and how to protect one's self from AIDS.)

Teaching materials:

1. News clipping on the AIDS situation in Thailand, "Thais fight AIDS," by the Population and Community Development Association"

2. Information sheets

3. Pictures about AIDS

Evaluation:

Observe the students' behaviour as follows:

- Participation in class activities
- Class discussions
- Cooperation within the group
- Presentation of group work

Suggested additional activities:

Sing the song, "AIDS."

ADDENDUM

AIDS Situation and its Effect on Thailand

AIDS is spreading rapidly in Thailand. People who are infected with HIV can be found in every province and in almost every amphur. They include people from all professions and from all walks of life, even newborn children and housewives. If we leave things the way they are right now, Thailand will face many problems in the future. Thailand is one of the many countries experiencing a very fast spread of AIDS, because of a complex network of causes for transmission. AIDS is spread through sexual contact with infected people, transfusion of HIV positive blood, and the sharing of needles with HIV carriers.

Prostitutes are considered the most dangerous group because they can spread AIDS more rapidly than other groups. Spouses can contract HIV from their partners. HIV infection is found among drug addicts, prisoners, young men 20-22 years old, labourers, government officials, employers of companies, and even monks.

It is obvious that the AIDS situation in Thailand has become increasingly crucial. There are approximately 300,000-400,000 people infected with HIV. The next problem the country will face is a drop in economic growth. Income from tourism and foreign investment may decrease or stop, because of the uncertainty of situation.

A part of the government budget will have to be allocated for the care and treatment of AIDS patient.

It is time for government and non-government agencies to work together to stop the spread of AIDS. AIDS is everyone's problem: all members of society have to help stop it before Thailand faces an economic disaster with large numbers of people dying in spite of the nation having no war or terrorist attacks.

Source: *Thais Fight AIDS, Population and Community Development Association.*

AIDS SONG

AIDS is a new disease. It destroys immunity.
The body is suddenly weak Because of its infection.
Finally emaciated No energy, just suffering
Saddening everyone. Listen to its prevention.
Use condoms during Sexual intercourse.
Have just one partner. Don't change ever.
If using a needle for drugs, AIDS will spread to
Whomever shares The same needle.
However dangerous AIDS is, You can't get it from breath.
Play and have fun And love with your heart.
If in doubt that You might have AIDS,
Go ahead and see a doctor. It's alright.

INFORMATION SHEET

Danger and Impact of AIDS on the Individual

1. Impact on Health:

A. Physical health: Suffering from the disease resulting in poor health until death.

B. Psychological health:

— No confidence n the, future. No sense of stability because of secretive life. Feeling uncertain about whether one's family, friends, and employer will accept his or her condition and not knowing whether one is dying and how long he or she will live. All these worries increase as time goes.

— Feeling one is losing out in many important things in life as a result of this illness, such as strength, sexual opportunities, and good looks, a role in society, and economic status.

2. Economic Impact:

— Expense of the treatment.

— Loss of income due to decreased ability to work.

— Rajection by employer and colleagues, leading to termination of employment.

— Inability to work and loss of income.

3. Social Impact:

— Being discriminated against by social and inability to live comfortably.

— Isolation from friends and family due to the risks of AIDS transmission. Limitation in living at home and in the larger society.

Danger and Impact of AIDS on Family

Economic Impact:

A. A family member's illness reduces the amount of labour available.

- A sick person works less or is not able to work at all.
- A sick person is the family's burden: other family members will have to spend time taking care of him/her instead of working.

B. Increased expense due to care and treatment.

Social Impact:

The transmission of AIDS creates barriers between the patient and the family. Other people in the family are afraid that they will be infected. They feel uncomfortable, both physically and emotionally about having to take care of the AIDS infected member of the family, AIDS brings tension and anxiety to the family.

Danaer and Impact of AIDS on Society (Country)

Economic Impact:

- Most AIDS patients are of working age. For these people to be unemployed or unable to work is a great loss to the country's economy.
- The patients' care and treatment are a big problem and burden for the country. The problem involves personnel and medical expense to provide care.
- Loss of human resources from the illness and death of young patients.

Social Impact:

- Fear caused by inadequate or inaccurate information about AIDS leads to discrimination againstAIDS patients, destroying good relations among people in the society. There will be suspicion and tension among the patients and other members of society. Living together will not be as peaceful as it used to be.

5

LOVE YOUR LIFE, DON'T EVEN CONSIDER GETTING AIDS

Content:

1. Avoiding sexual relations and not sharing needles and sharp objects with people who have AIDS will help protect you from AIDS.

2. The ability to choose to do the right things can help reduce the risk of AIDS.

Objectives:

To be able to:

- *identify risky behaviour that can lead to AIDS transmission;*

- *give examples of situations that may lead to risky sexual behaviour resulting in HIV infection;*

- *give guidelines on how to behave to avoid contracting AIDS.*

Teaching activities:

1. Sing the "AIDS" song.

2. Discuss the content of the song. Ask the students what information they get from it.

Answers: - Cause (virus that destroys the body's immune system)

- Symptoms (weak, emaciated, no energy)

- Prevention (use a condom when having sexual intercourse, do not share needles for drugs, see a doctor if showing probable symptoms)

- AIDS cannot be transmitted through the breath or through playing together.

3. Summarize the information from the song. Discuss how AIDS is actually transmitted.

   AIDS cannot be transmitted through mosquitoes, eating together, swimming in the same pool, or sharing a bathroom.

4. Have students study prepared poster, "Which is NOT a Mode of AIDS Transmission?" Discuss and summarize.

5. Ask students to give examples of situations that may lead to a sexual relation risky for contracting AIDS.

   - Being invited by a stranger

   - Being alone with a member of the opposite sex

   - Seeking sexual experience from a prostitute, etc.

Have a class discussion on how to behave, and have students record it in their notebook.

6. Summarize the above discussion.

Teaching materials:

1. Chart of "AIDS" song
2. AIDS poster

Evaluation:

Observe students' cooperation in answering questions and their interest in particiı ating in activities.

Suggested additional activities:

1. Create a bulletin board
2. Make a chart showing risky sexual behaviour.
3. Develop a survey questionnaire to assess attitudes of people in the community towards behaviour that risks contracting AIDS.

ACTIVITIES

Questionnaire

Knowledge about AIDS

Statment	Yes	No
1. Have you ever shared your toothbrush?	....	....
2. Have you ever received blood transfusion?	....	....
3. Have you ever been to a prostitute?	....	....
4. Have you ever shared your injection needles?	....	....
5. Have you ever used a needle for a tattoo and for piercing your ears?	....	....
6. Have you ever shared sharp objects?	....	....

6

IF THERE IS LIFE, THERE IS HOPE

CONTENT:

People who are infected with HIV and AIDS can live for another 5-8 years if they take good care of themselves.

OBJECTIVES:

To be able to:

- *tell how people with HIV and people with AIDS should take care of themselves*
- *describe the Dharma for family life*
- *give suggestions on how to lead a good life*

Teaching activities:

1. Hand out information sheet, "Life Accident" by Dr. Nopporn,

MD. Discuss and ask questions relating to the following topics:

- What are the feelings of a person infected with HIV?
- Is the person behaving properly or not? Why?
- If you were infected with HIV, how would you behave?
- Summarize proper behaviour.

2. Read and do role playing of the situation of "Ms. Yensabai" and analyze it, using the following topics:

- Why did Ms. Yensabai want to commit suicide?
- Was she right in thinking suicide was a solution?
- How would you help and advise Ms. Yensabai solve the problem?

Summarize and make suggestions on what an HIV-infected person and an AIDS patient should do.

3. Ask students to quote the Dharma for family life and to apply it in daily life, namely, the Dharma for lay people and the contentment of a married person.

Dharma for Lay People

- Truthfulness and intention to do good
- Suppression of desire to do evil
- Patience and perseverance in doing good
- Discarding evil ideas and evil deeds

Contentment of a Married Person

- Contentment comes from prosperity
- Contentment comes from spending one's earnings
- Contentment comes from not being in debt
- Contentment comes from harmless behaviour

Teaching materials:

1. Information sheet: "Life Accident"
2. The story of "Ms. Yensabai"

Evaluation:

1. Observe students' participation in and attention to the discussion and debate.

2. Their courage in acting in the role play.

Suggested additional activities:

1. Collect articles on AIDS.

2. Show a video tape on AIDS.

3. Practice meditation and follow the Dharma.

4. Have a debate on the topic, "People with AIDS are more deserving of disgust than sympathy".

INFORMATION SHEET

Life Accident

Dear Dr. Nopporn:

I am a regular follower of your column in the Daily News. I was born in a poor farming family but we were happy. I am better educated than my siblings because I received a scholarship. My parents were very pleased about that. Since I graduated and started working, I have been sending some money to my poor parents. In my life, I don't want anything other than for my parents to live a more comfortable live.

Now I am very upset and sad because I have been infected by HIV. I have tried to cope with it by reading the Dharma. I am not going to kill myself. I don't blame myself, or my friends, or the social environment. I think it must be my karma from the former life. I had three blood tests and the doctor has confirmed that I am HIV positive. I think I am in phase two. I had a severe weight loss from 60 kilograms to 50 kilograms. I have experienced a number of symptoms such as fever, poor appetite, diarrhoea, and thrush on my tongue. I have been hiding this from my family and colleagues. I have been trying to exercise and eat plenty of food, but I feel weaker everyday. Mentally,

I feel strong enough but I am very concerned about my parents and my poor family. I have been supporting them. My younger siblings and my nieces and nephews are still in school. Every month I hardly get to spend my own salary.

I think my life boat is sinking. Within one to two years, I will be bombarded by different diseases but I will try to move along in my life boat as far as I can. I am certain that I will not kill myself because my parents will be most upset by that. I have been studying the Dharma.

I would like to ask you to help find somebody who would help my family. I know they would face difficulties after I die. If there is such a kind person, I will be happy to meet you and show you the results of my blood tests, but I don't want anybody in the mass media to know about this because I am afraid my parents will find out. I hope you understand and I hope there will be people who want to help my family.

I don't drink and I don't smoke. I have been to a prostitute four times in my whole life and I am HIV positive. I'd like to call it a life accident.

From a son who is always grateful to his parents

ACTIVITIES

Dramatization/Role Play

Ms. Yensabai

Characters: Ms. Yensabai

Mother -Doctor

Narrator: Yensabai was a beautiful woman who used to be a prostitute in Pattaya. After she quit her job as a prostitute, she went back to her home. Her personality had changed from being cheerful to being introverted, quiet, sad, and worried. She was pale and in poor health. Her mother felt concerned, so she took Yensabai to see a doctor at the hospital.

Doctor: Khun Yensabai, please relax and don't worry too much. The result from the blood tests indicates that you are infected by the AIDS virus. It is a fatal disease that is incurable.

Yensabai: (Frightened and upset) There is absolutely no cure?

Doctor: I'm sorry, no. However, you can live longer if you take good care of your physical and mental health. During the period when there are no symptoms, you can lead a normal life, but you must remember not to have sexual relations with anybody so that you don't transmit the disease to others. Please follow my advice.

Narrator: Yensabai and her mother went home. Yensabai was so upset that she wanted to kill herself. Her mother calmed her down.

Mother: Killing yourself is not a good solution. There are ways for one to lead a happy life before one dies. We have to fight. You can still be helpful to your parents and society; for example, you can advise your friends and your family how to avoid contracting the infection. The doctor also said you can avoid spreading the disease. If you stay home and accept the reality and calm your mind, you can live a peaceful life.

Yensabai: Yes, mother. I will try to follow your advice.

Narrator: Yensabai has been following her mother's advice, trying to keep a strong mind and a determination to live by applying the Dharma to her life.

7

HAVE EMPATHY TOWARDS OTHERS

CONTENT:

People who are infected with HIV and AIDS should be treated humanely and with empathy.

Objectives:

To be able to:

- develop empathy towards people who are infected with HIV and AIDS;
- provide help to AIDS patients as needed;
- advise AIDS patients on how to take care of themselves;
- explain how to live with people who are infected with HIV and AIDS.

Teaching activities:

1. Organize a debate on "AIDS Patients are more Disgusting than Pitiful";

2. Read "A Viewpoint from Damri" (Fai's spouse);

3. Discuss how to live with people who are infected with HIV and AIDS relating to these topics:

- Providing help
- Having empathy
- Providing emotional support
- No discrimination

4. Summarize and record comments

Teaching materials:

1. "A Viewpoint from Damri"

2. Debate topic

3. AIDS printed materials

Evaluation:

Observe students' behaviour in the following areas:

- Participation in class activities
- Attention and interest in seeking more information
- Providing good reasons in group discussion

ADDENDUM

A Viewpoint from Damri

"It has been more than a year since I have been infected with HIV. My body is still functioning normally and we live our life with love and understanding, taking good care of each other. There are also people from the Association who help us and give us moral support. Whenever Fai has to give a lecture somewhere, I am always there driving her around.

"We can still fight to live because we have the will power. If we think we want to live, we have to make up our mind to be strong. If we feel discouraged, we will deteriorate quickly. It probably takes months to accept the situation and it depends on the individual.

"Fai's work is very useful in helping people understand about the disease and its prevention. However, there is a big disadvantage. The more people know about us, the more difficulty we face. Nobody knows what it is like in my family. We have an anxious home; everybody in my family is worried that he will lose his job because of us, just like what happened to Khun Cha-on. We received a number of threatening phone calls. It is very hard to live peacefully. The situation has improved a little lately.

"A lot of people in my neighbourhood look at me as if I were a monster. They look down on me and express their disgust. I try not to think too much about it. Some people who are nicer smile at me and ask how I am."

Source: Klai Mo magazine, No 4, April 1992.

8

KNOWING OUR BODIES

CONTENT:

When we enter the teenage years, our bodies experience physical and psychological changes.

OBJECTIVES:

To be able to:

- *describe physical and psychological changes during adolescence;*
- *state problems arising from inappropriate sexual behaviour;*
- *describe how to build a healthy body and a healthy mind.*

Teaching activities:

1. Have students study charts of the human body at different ages (age 10-15 years);

2. Discuss and compare physical development at various stages:

   - Body proportion (size)
   - Weight
   - Height
   - Physical changes (organs)

3. Divide students into groups to study the information sheets regarding teenage development in various aspects.

   - Physical
   - Emotional
   - Social

4. Ask students to give examples of teenage behaviour

   - Cultivating curiosity with the desire to learn
   - Respecting others
   - Not hanging around
   - Using free time effectively
   - Being responsible
   - Going out at night
   - Sniffing glue and smoking cigarettes
   - Dressing according to new fashions
   - Acting like adults etc.

5. Have students identify inappropriate types of sexual behaviour and analyze their disadvantages.

Inappropriate sexual behaviour	Disadvantages
1. Acting like adults	1. Being deceived 2. Spending money wastefully 3. Being raped 4. Leading to premature sex
2. Going out at night	1. Poor health 2. Waste of money 3. Being deceived 4. Being abducted

6. Help students summarize and make up guidelines for maintaining a healthy body and a healthy mind, such as:

- Regular exercise
- Effective use of spare time
- Keeping a clean body
- Accepting physical changes, etc.

Teaching activities:

1. Pictures of people of different ages
2. Information sheets
3. Printed materials about AIDS and teenagers

Evaluation:

Observe students' behaviour, taking into account their participation in class activities, class discussion, and in making up guidelines for healthy behaviour.

Suggested additional activities:

1. Carry out some useful activities such as planting trees, cleaning up the school compound, etc.

2. Have students record their own physical, emotional, and social development, including height, weight, the ability to get along with others, and any other changes. This may be done for a month or a semester.

9

A CLOSELY-KNIT FAMILY CAN EASILY FIGHT AIDS

CONTENT:

Love and understanding in the family are a good foundation for preventing AIDS

OBJECTIVES:

To be able to:

- *state the different roles of family members;*
- *express bonding between parents and children;*
- *state the impact upon one's family when someone in the family contracts the AIDS virus;*
- *suggest solutions to family problems.*

Teaching activities:

1. Sing the song "Family Fights AIDS"

2. Discuss the content of the song. Ask students the following questions:

   - What does the song talk about?
   - Why are love and bonding important?
   - How can warmth in one's family help prevent AIDS?

Summarize the discussion and point out the roles of different family members and the importance of love, understanding, and bonding among parents and children.

3. Divide students into groups to study the story "Prapai's Life" and involve students in discussion after reading.

4. Each group representative reports his group's work to the class.

5. Help the students summarize the following topics:

   - The role of family
   - The importance of bonding between parents and children in solving problems and preventing AIDS.

Teaching materials:

1. Chart of "Family Fights AIDS" song
2. Printed materials about AIDS
3. Discussion topics

Evaluation:

Observe students' participation in class discussion, cooperation with others and attention.

Suggested Additional Activities:

1. Draw a picture of a happy family.
2. Collect news picture about good families
3. Organize a slogan contest.

ACTIVITIES

Prapai's Life

Prapai grew up in a small, poor family in the country. When she finished sixth grade, she came to Bangkok to look for work. Because of her good looks she got a job as a waitress in a restaurant. After working there for a while, a man showed interest in her. Prapai was lonely and naive; she dreamed of having a nice family of her own. It didn't take long before Prapai felt close to the man. He asked to take her home to ask for her hand from her parents. On the way he asked Prapai to stop at a building because he had business there. However, he disappeared and a woman who turned out to be the owner of the building showed up. Prapai then knew that she had been deceived into entering a brothel by her boyfriend.

At the brothel Prapai was forced to receive clients. She was hurt both physically and emotionally, living in a dirty and cramped brothel and seeing all kinds of men. Four months later Prapai became pregnant. The pimp, seeing that Prapai had been sick a lot and could no longer bring in a good income, gave Prapai one hundred baht to go home.

Prapai came home battered. She told the whole story to her mother. Her mother took her to see a doctor. After listening to her story, the doctor ordered some blood tests and found that Prapai was infected with the AIDS virus.

Prapai's family had nobody to turn to, so the doctor advised Prapai to stay at an emergency home. There she received sympathy and help, which enabled her to continue living.

Even though Prapai lost her child to AIDS when he was only a year old, she spent the last part of her life at the emergency home. She helped others in every way she could. She used her small income to buy gifts for her parents and nieces and nephews when she visited them. Sometimes she lectured about her life to try to get others to understand people who had AIDS using her life story as a reminder for the rest of the world.

Involve the students in discussion relating to the following questions:

1. Question: How do you feel about Prapai's life?

   Answer: Sympathetic.

2. Question: Why did Prapai have to come to Bangkok?

   Answers:

   - Her parents are poor, and she needed to work.
   - Life was diffcult.
   - Her parents sent her there to earn some money.

3. Question: Why did Prapai become a prostitute?

   Answers: - She was naive, which caused her to be deceived.

   - She was forced into it. - She wanted to make more money.

4. Question: Should parents send their children to work in Bangkok while they are still young Qust out of 6th grade)? Why?

   Answers: No, they shouldn't because they can be easily deceived and may end up like Prapai.

5. Question: When you grow up and become parents yourselves, what should be your role after your children finish their elementary education?

   Answers: - Support them in continuing their education.

   - Keep them near me and let them learn about life for a while.
   - When they are old enough to work far away, make sure that the work will not lead them to the same fate as Prapai's. (Use the form below to provide additional answers) .

6. Question: If someone in your family became infected with the AIDS virus, what might be some of the problems and what would your solutions be? Use the form below.

ACTIVITIES

PROBLEM SOLVING

Problem ....

....

Impact ....

....

Solution ....

....

....

Options   Evaluation of Options

....

advantages	disadvantages	practical	unpractical
....	....	....	....
....	....	....	....
....	....	....	....
....	....	....	....
....	....	....	....

ADDENDUM

Family Fights AIDS

Words by Jirapong Khamphiw

Tune from Dek Pump

(Summary:) The Thai family is good because we have father, mother, and brothers and sisters. We love each other and we are united to do the right things according to Thai culture. Parents need to have love and bonding as power for fighting AIDS. AIDS is so serious a disease that one should not contract it. No other words can be said if you have AIDS, except death.

10

NIT-NOI GOES TO THE DOCTOR

Content:

To maintain good health, one needs to take good care of all body parts. This can also prevent AIDS infection.

Objectives:

To be able to:

- *tell the importance of each body part;*
- *take proper care of all body parts regularly;*
- *identify behaviour that is not consistent with sexual health.*

Teaching activities:

1. Conduct a health assessment activity by having students examine each other (hands, hair, mouth, ears, eyes, teeth, etc:)

2. Discuss the following topics:

   - What causes body parts to be dirty?

- The results of not taking proper care of the body.
- Diseases in different body parts (with emphasis on sexual organs).

3. Have students read "Nit-Noi Went to see a Doctor." Engage the students in discussion relating to the following topics:

   - Why did Nit-noi have to see a doctor?
   - What is the cause of her illness?
   - How can it be prevented?

4. Help students develop some guidelines for proper care of sexual organs.

5. Discuss certain types of behaviour that are inconsistent with sexual health, such as:

   - Improper cleaning of sexual organs after elimination or after menstruation
   - Premature sex
   - Not using condoms during sexual intercourse
   - Using condoms incorrectly etc.

6. Summarize the guidelines and have the students write them in their notebooks.

Teaching materials:

1. Students' bodies, pictures, and models
2. The story, "Nit-noi Goes to the doctor"
3. Pictures about different diseases in different parts of body

Evaluation:

Observe students' participation in class activities, attention, and reasoning in class discussion .

Suggested additional activities:

1. Write up slogans on how to keep the body clean.
2. Conduct research in the library.

ADDENDUM

Nit-noi Goes to the Doctor

One day Nit-noi, who was five, was taken to see a doctor by her mother Nit-noi had been having foul-smelling vaginal discharge. The doctor thought that some feces might have got into her vagina due to improper cleaning. The doctor gave the mother the following advice on how to clean the private area properly:

- After each defecation, wipe off any feces, and then rinse the area with clean water.

- Wash the vaginal area with clean water after urination.

Nit-noi's mother thanked the doctor and then asked "Do boys need to wash after each urination like girls?"

The doctor answered, "No, they don't. Boys may develop some inflammation if their foreskin is longer than normal. This can cause urine to accumulate at the tip of the penis which will become reddened and painful when the boy urinates. However, both boys and girls should learn how to take proper care of their sexual organs on a regular basis."

11

MEET IN THE MIDDLE

CONTENT:

Proper understanding of human sexual nature leads to happy living in the society.

OBJECTIVES:

To be able to:

- *give examples of appropriate sexual adjustment;*
- *give examples of sexual values in society;*
- *evaluate and choose sexual values correctly.*

Teaching activities:

1. Divide into groups and have three boys debate against three girls on the topic, "Women's Love is Truer than Men's."

2. Discuss differences in values between men and women.

   2.1 Sexual love

Men - begin with desire and slowly change into love and affection.

Women - begin with love and affection before having desire.

2.2. Leadership

Men - Front legs

Women - Hind legs

3. Summarize from the discussion concerning values in Thai society.

- Men with many wives are considered capable.
- Women with many husbands are considered bad.
- The myth that sexua! ability depends on the size of the penis and duration of intercourse.

4. Have students read the following article:

By nature men and women have the same desires, but our society does not allow the same means of expressing them. Men have greater freedom of expression and it is considered necessary for them to express their desires. Women cannot do that, perhaps because a woman has the responsibility of bearing a child and cannot refuse to be a man's wife after becoming pregnant; whereas men do not have to take any responsibility for pregnancy. That is why parents in the old days tended to keep their daughters away from men and repressed them, thinking that if there were no male stimulation, their daughters would be careful and no untoward incident would occur.

In Western society, the value of virginity has greatly changed. Women lose their virginity early on. It does not matter if men care about virginity because women do not worry about it. There is no winner and no loser. Sex is considered a mutual activity with both sides neither gaining nor losing. This change comes mostly from women.

In the past, women were not self-sufficient, and could not support themselves throughout their lives. Today women are professionals, capable of taking care of themselves. After finishing their education, they look for a place to live alone, either out of preference or out of necessity. They learn to take care of themselves at a young age. Some of them have to leave home in the provinces to go to school in Bangkok. After college they find work in Bangkok and never return home to live. They have to make their own decisions. Their living arrangements allow them to fulfill their desire for men conveniently. Women and men may live together for a while before marriage to find out whether they can share their life in the future.

Discuss the article.

5. Summarize together the desirable values:

   5.1 Family problems are an important matter that affects all of us. Some of the problems are about earning a living; others are about love affairs, with either the husband or the wife involved in an affair.

The basis of this problem comes from sexual inequality, such as:

- Perception of the wife as an emotional receptacle:
- Not listening to each other, etc.

6. Help students summarize values that need to be inculcated, such as
   - Listen and accept the others' opinion. If there is any problem, talk to one another.
   - Care for one another. - Respect each other.
   - Be honest and faithful to one another. - Be tolerant, etc.
7. Show pictures of warm and loving families

Teaching materials:

1. Debate topic, "Women's Love is Truer than Men's"
2. Reading materials about Dharma
3. Pictures of warm and loving families

Evaluation:

Observe students' participation in class activities, cooperation between groups, and class discussion.

Suggested additional activities:

1. Draw pictures of warm and loving families.
2. Draw a chart of the Dharma concerning family.
3. Essay contest about the family such as "The Family I Want"

12

WE DON'T WANT TO CONTRACT AIDS

CONTENTS:

1. AIDS is a fatal communicable disease. It is incurable and there & is no vaccine to prevent it.

2. People who are HIV positive will develop AIDS within 5-8 years.

3. People who have AIDS usually develop secondary infections due to a weakened immune system.

OBJECTIVES:

To be able to:

- *state the rationale for studying about AIDS*
- *give the definition of AIDS*
- *describe the source of infection and its transmission*
- *describe its symptoms*
- *gather more information conceming AIDS.*

LEARNING ACTIVITIES:

1. Assign two or three students to read news clippings concerning AIDS, after which the whole class should discuss and summarize the content regarding the adverse effects of AIDS upon oneself, one's family and the society as a whole.

2. Discuss the reasons why students need to learn about AIDS and summarize the discussion.

3. Assess students' attitudes towards being HIV positive and having AIDS.

4. Divide students into four groups to play "WHO AM I?"

5. Have a representative from each group report to the class what they have learned from playing the game.

6. Have the students study prepared documents or watch AIDS video tape.

7. Each group is given a work sheet with a list of activities to complete.

8. The whole class draws conclusions from different work sheets on the following topics:

   - *Why do we need to learn about AIDS?*
   - *What does AIDS mean?*
   - *The cause of AIDS and its transmission.*
   - *The difference between being HIV positive and having AIDS.*

Teaching materials:

1. Newspapers, pamphlets and AIDS video tape.
2. Game "Who am I?"
3. Worksheets.
4. Worksheet- We Don't Want to Contract AIDS.

Evaluation:

1. Observe students' participation in group activities and class discussion.

2. Check student worksheets for correct usage and acceptable answers.

Suggested additional activities:

1. Students are encouraged to research in the school library or at the book corner in the classroom.

2. Put up a bulletin board on the topic of AIDS.

3. Encourage students to follow the news about AIDS from newspapers, radio and television.

ACTIVITIES

GAME: WHO AM I ?

Cut this sheet into strips and put into an envelope. Make as many copies as needed. Each group of students tries to put the puzzle together as fast as possible. The first to complete will get a prize.

AIDS

HIV snfection

Hidden within the body

It can be transmitted even if the person is strong and without any symptoms.

Secondary infections

Duration of 5-8 years or longer

Infected person

The person dies.

ACTIVITIES

Activity Worksheet

Directions:

Select a leader and a secretary for each group before you start. Then follow the directions below:

1. The group leader reads the following questions to the group:
   - Why do we need to learn about AIDS?
   - What does AIDS mean?
   - What is the cause of AIDS and its transmission
   - What is the difference between being HIV positive and having AIDS?
2. Group discussion is carried on to answer the questions.
3. The secretary records the answers on the paper provided and hands it in to the teacher.

Answer Sheet

ACTIVITIES

Summary Form: We don't want to contract AIDS

Group ------------------------------------

Group Member

1. ------------------------------ group leader
2. ------------------------------ member
3. ------------------------------ member
4. ------------------------------ secretary

1. Why do we need to learn about AIDS?

   ----

2. What does AIDS mean?

   ----

3. What is the cause of AIDS and its transmission?

   ----

4. What is the difference between being HIV-positive and having AIDS?

13

AIDS IS PREVENTABLE

CONTENT:

AIDS is preventable. A person who has AIDS should take good care of him/herself to slow down its progress. People in society should be understanding and offer help.

OBJECTIVES:

To be able to:

- *name sources of HIV;*
- *describe how the virus is transmitted to the human body;*
- *explain how people with AIDS should take care of themselves;*
- *describe prevention and AIDS transmission;*
- *express empathy and try to offer help to infected people.*

Learning Activities:

1. Review by asking questions and have the class listen to students read news clippings about people with AIDS.

2. Discuss physical and psychological conditions of AIDS patients.

3. Divide the students into four groups. Have each group study the following case studies;

   — Cha-on Sualoom who contracted AIDS from blood transfusion, story from Thai Rath, September 9, 1989

   — Magic Johnson, famous American basketball player

4. Students in each group discuss their feelings and how they would treat people who are HIV positive and people with AIDS.

5. Watch a video tape on AIDS or read about AIDS patients and answer the following questions:

   — What are the sources of the AIDS virus and how is it transmitted to the human body?

   — How should an infected person take care of himself?

   — How should you treat a person who is HIV positive or a person with AIDS and his family?

6. Give students additional information about blood screening before blood transfusion and where to obtain blood tests for AIDS.

Teaching materials:

1. Newspapers
2. Video tape about AIDS
3. Case studies

Evaluation:

1. Observe class participation
2. Check student assignment for language usage and clarity

Suggested additional activities:

1. AIDS picture scrapbook

2. AIDS news clippings scrapbook

3. Write a composition on one's feelings towards AIDS patients

4. Organize AIDS activities such as slogan contest, drawing contest, debate and an exhibition.

ACTIVITIES

CASE STUDY

Directions:

1. Select group leaders and group secretaries.
2. The case study is read to the group by the group leader.
3. Group discussion on the case study.
4. Group secretary records the answers on the paper provided.

An excerpt from an interview with Cha-on Sualoom from Thai Rath newspaper, September 9, 1989

"My family and I have suffered a great deal since I contracted AIDS. My oldest son, a head mechanic in a well known company, was forced to quit his job. The same happened to the other two who were working at a battery factory, when they learned that I had AIDS. My youngest child is now 8 and is going to school. I can't afford to pay for my children's education. When my children went out to look for a house to rent, people refused to rent their houses when they learned they were my children. I, myself, have to keep moving. I cannot stay with my children because I don't want to cause them any trouble. Please tell the public that I am the only one with AIDS and that no one else in my family has it. Please have some compassion."

Answer the following questions;

1. What is your feeling towards Mr. Cha-on Sualoom?

2. If you lived in the same community with him, how would you treat him and his family?

3. Do you think it is Mr. Cha-on's fault that he got AIDS?

4. If you were Mr. Cha-on, how would you take care of yourself?

Case study; Magic Johnson

Answer the following questions:

1. How do you feel about Magic Johnson?

....

....

....

2. Why is Magic Johnson infected with AIDS?

....

....

....

3. When he knew he had contracted the AIDS virus, how did he feel and how did he take care of himself?

....

....

....

4. If you were Magic Johnson, how would you lead a happy life in your society?

....

....

....

14

AIDS IS A DANGER TO LIFE AND SOCIETY

CONTENT:

AIDS is a fatal, transmited disease that brings about a serious impact upon the socio-economic well-being of society. We should be aware of the importance of preventing and controlling AIDS.

OBJECTIVES:

To be able to:

- develop an awareness that AIDS is dangerous and is everyone's problem
- analyze the impact of AIDS upon human life and the society
- draw personal conclusion regarding the treat of AIDS on one's life and the society.

Learning activifes:

1. Divide the students into two groups. Each group sends a

representative to play the game-Ma Tam Nat, a matching game.

2. Review previous lessons after the game.

3. Divide the students into four groups. Each group receives a worksheet with a list of activities to do.

4. Group representatives give a report of group dicussion on the impact of AIDS upon individuals, family, and community.

5. Students and teacher come to the following conclusion:

   AIDS is a serious, socially transmited disease. An infected person usually dis at an early age. Most people who are HIV-positive and develop AIDS are still considerably young and, therefore, at an age where they could conthbute to the socio-economic development of the country. It is important that we work together to control AIDS.

6. From activity 5, each gnup has to come up withh a proper slogan on the impact of AIDS on human life, socity and the economy.

Teaching materials:

1. Game-Ma Tam Nat

2. Worksheet - AIDS is dangerous to life and detrimental to society.

3. Examples of AIDS slogans

4. Information papers on AIDS with an emphasis on the high cost of treatment and loss of incorne and human resource.

Evaluation:

1. Observe the students' attention, cooperation and participation, and their ability to discuss, reason and summarize the concepts.

2. Assess their understanding from written slogans.

Suggested additional activities:

1. Ask the students to write an essay or a short story about the danger of AIDS to develop an awareness of AIDS as everyone's problem, one that everybody must help to prevent and control.

2. Arrange a bulletin board exhibition on the danger of AIDS, using slogans and reports from group work, essays and stories.

3. Organize a campaign against AIDS by posting slogans in the school and in public places in the community.

ACTIVITIES

GAME: MA TAM NAT

Materials:

1. Flash cards with these words: AIDS, probable symptoms, transmission, and prevention.

2. Flash cards of phrases:

   - via blood and blood transfusion
   - sexual intercourse
   - from pregnant mother to her foetus
   - sharing the same needle for drug injection
   - sexual promiscuity
   - avoid coming into contact with somebody else's blood
   - if accidentally in contact with somebody else's blood or body fluid, immediately wash the affected area with soap and water
   - do not share sharp objects with others
   - blood tests before getting married
   - enlarged lymph nodes

- chronic fever without known cause
- drastic weight loss
- chronic thrushes in oral cavity
- having herpes on and off
- chronic diarrhoea

Teacher preparation:

1. Place flash cards of AIDS, probable symptoms, transmission, and prevention into different columns on the board.

2. Mix up the rest of the cards and leave them on the front desk.

Using the same kind of activity:

1. Divide the students into two groups.

2. Pair students from these two groups.

3. Start the game with the first pair of students by having a student from the first group pick up a card from the desk, read it aloud and ask a student from the other group to which column the phrase belongs. The other student must place the card under the right column on the board.

4. The game proceeds in the same manner with a student from the second group picking up a card.

Scoring:

1. One point is given for each correct answer.
2. No more than five seconds are given to answer the question.

ACTIVITIES

Worksheet

Directions:

1. Select group leaders and group secretaries.

2. Study "AIDS IS DANGEROUS TO LIFE AND DETRIMENTAL TO SOCIETY".

3. Discuss, analyze, and write a summary on the impacts of AIDS upon individuals, families, communities and the country.

4. Send a group representative to present the group's work to the class.

AIDS IS DANGEROUS TO LIFE AND DETRIMENTAL TO SOCIETY

Why is AIDS dangerous?

AIDS is dangerous because once a person is infected, he cannot be cured. The person will suffer until he dies. There is a wrong impression that AIDS is easily transmitted. AIDS cannot be transmitted through casual contact and AIDS is preventable. Society is severely affected by the spread of AIDS, especially by the high cost of treatment. The infected person may feel frightened and hopeless and may commit suicide. If the spread of AIDS continues at the present rate, a lot of people will die from it within the next ten years. People's behaviour and way of life will change. There will be an increase in the use of condoms, more discrimination against homosexuality, decrease in drug use fewer men going to prostitutes, and probably many requests for blood tests before marriage.

AIDS can slow development and obstruct economic progress because the people who die of AIDS are usually young. They are an important resources in developing the country. The remaining children and elderly would not be able to bring about development as well. Besides, part of the country's resource would have to be allocated for treatment, prevention and education Industrial development would face a number of obstacles: fewer foreign investments, Thai exports facing tough barriers, Thai labour facing discrimination in overseas employment, fewer tourists would come to Thailand, and there would be a general slowdown of economic expansion.

Is it about time for us to fight against AIDS?

Compiled from "QUESTIONS AND ANSWERS ABOUT AIDS" by Dr. Sathaporn Manasthit

15

PROTECT YOURSELF FROM AIDS

CONTENT:

1. Remarkable changes occur, both physically and mentally, during pre-adolescence.

2. Self-control over sexual behaviour can prevent AIDS.

OBJECTIVES:

To be able to:

— *describe physical and mental changes during pre-teen period and sexual and psychological development of teenage boys and girls.*

— *identify problems and effects of inappropriate sexual behaviour.*

— *assess and make appropriate decisions to avoid unhealthy and inappropriate sexual behaviour.*

Teaching activities:

1. Show two pictures to students, one of young children and the other of teenagers. Have students compare differences in physical development, including body proportion, height, and changes in sexual organs and sex hormones.

2. Divide the students into groups to read an article, "Emotional and Mental Development of Teenagers". Then carry on a group discussion on the following topics:

   — Teenagers' emotional changes: give some examples.

   — Suggestions about the sexual and emotional development of teenagers.

   — A report of the group discussions is presented to the class by a representative from each group. The teacher helps the class carry on the discussion and draw conclusions.

3. Ask to students to have some examples a teenage behaviour, such as:

- going out at night
- playing sports
- smoking cigarette and drinking
- interest in the opposite sex and acting like grown ups, etc.

4. Ask the students to pick out some of the undesirable behaviour mentioned and state their negative effects.

Behaviour	*Bad effects*
1. Going out at night	1. Being deceived
2.	2. Poor health
	3. Getting infected

5. Help the students summarize the kinds of behaviour that lead to the risk of contracting AIDS.

6. Divide the students into four groups to work on the worksheet and discuss types of behaviour that risk contracting AIDS, such as not knowing how to say "no", or being too easy and too casual.

7. Each group sends a group representative to report to the class.

8. Help the students draw up some guidelines to avoid sexual relationships before the right time, such as:

- do not drink with or accept a drink from people you don't know

- avoid being alone with someone in an isolated area

- do not go out with a member of the opposite sex alone

- know how to say "no" when being encouraged to do something inappropriate

- when having sexual desire, learn how to help oneself, which is safer than going to a prostitute or getting involved in premature sexual relationship.

Teaching materials:

1. Pictures
2. Reading materials
3. Worksheet

Evaluation:

Observe student participation, co-operation, and reasoning in group discussions.

ACTIVITIES

Activity Worksheet

Directions:

1. Select group leaders and group secretaries
2. The group leader reads the assigned reading to the group
3. Carry on group discussion
4. The group secretary records the group discussion.

Daeng is a friend of Peung's brother. Peung is in Grade 6. One day Daeng asks Peung to go to a park with him. Peung agrees to go without telling her parents. They walk hand in hand. At the end Daeng takes Peung to his relative's house. His relative is out of town.

Discussion topics:

1. Do you agree with Peung's behaviour?

2. Do you think Peung's behaviour can accidentally lead to sexual relationship and to potential AIDS infection?

3. If you were Peung, what would you do?

16

LEADING A GOOD LIFE THAT IS FREE FROM AIDS

CONTENT:

Loving one's self and valuing one's life leads to a quality of life that is free from AIDS.

OBJECTIVES:

To be able to:

— *give examples of social sexual ethics and appropriate sexual values*

— *explain differences in boys' and girls' interest in the opposite sex*

— *describe relationships that are free from AIDS*

Teaching activities:

1. To review, ask the students what kind of relationships can lead to an AIDS infection.

Answers may include; Going out with friends at night, drinking, using drugs, and going out alone with a member of the opposite sex.

2. Divide students into four or five groups to study a case study in the worksheet. Discuss and draw conclusions.

3. Class discussion and conclusion:

Men and women have different ideas of and interests in the opposite sex. Men tend to mix feelings of love and desire together (sexual need). Women seem to develop their love from admiration and faith and consider certain men as close friends (emotional need). A sexual encounter can occur when one side assumes the other side shares the same feeling. Both men and women should learn how to protect themselves from unintended sexual relationships. To stay free from AIDS, people should learn to use condoms and conduct themselves according to acceptable sexual values.

4. Assign students to prepare self-evaluation forms.

Teaching materials:

Case study: Life Path

Evaluation:

1. Observe student participation and reasoning in group discussion.
2. Check students' self-evaluation forms.
3. Students make their own choices.

Suggested additional activities:

1. AIDS bulletin board

2. Make a scrap book on appropriate and inappropriate teenage behaviour with captions and suggested acceptable behaviour.

ACTIVITIES

Worksheet

Directions:

Select group leader and group secretary. Then follow the steps below:

1. Group leader hands out a worksheet for the case study, Life Path, to each member.
2. Read and discuss the case study according to the following topics:

    1. What kind of a person is Tong?

        ....

        ....

    2. What kind of a person is Oy?

        ....

        ....

    3. Do you think Tong's and Oy's behaviour is proper or not? Explain.

        ....

        ....

    4. Do you think there is any difference between a man's love and a woman's love? Why?

        ....

        ....

    5. How should you conduct yourself in a male-female relationship in order to protect yourself from AIDS?

        ....

        ....

Case Study: Life Path

Tong had been skipping school every day. He and some of his friends had been using drugs and visiting prostitutes. He could not keep up with his classes. It was close to the final exams, and Tong was concerned that he would fail. He tried to borrow notes from friends, but everybody refused to help except Oy, who felt sorry for him. Oy let him borrow her notebooks and helped him review the lessons. They became very close.

When Tong and Oy learned that they both passed their exams, they decided to celebrate in Tong's room, where they had sexual intercourse.

Sometime later, Tong began to feel weak; he also had chronic low grade fever. He went to see a doctor. After a series of blood tests, Tong was found to have the AIDS virus and AIDS-related symptoms. In the meantime, Oy was feeling nauseous and vomiting and had to see a doctor. She was three months pregnant.

ACTIVITIES

Self-Evaluation Form

Directions: Mark an × in the appropriate column that appropriately describes your behaviour or attitude

No.	Behaviour	Yes	No
1.	I go out alone with a member/members of the opposite sex.	....	....
2.	I go out at night with a member/members of the opposite sex.	....	....
3.	I associate with bad people.	....	....
4.	I have been involved in sex prematurely.	....	....
5.	I have respect for the opposite sex.	....	....
6.	When invited to visit a prostitute, I usually agree to go.	....	....
7.	I am mindful of my actions.	....	....
8.	I dress modestly.	....	....
9.	I know how to say no when asked to do something wrong.	....	....

10. I am not sexually promiscuous.	....	....
11. I don't take drugs.	....	....
12. I use condoms.	....	....
13. I am reserved.	....	....
14. I skip school a lot.	....	....
15. I have had boyfriends or girifriends too soon.	....	....
16. When I experience a sexual desire, I play sports or engage in diversionary activities.	....	....

....

Signature ....

17

HAPPY FAMILY, FREE FROM AIDS

CONTENT:

Before starting a family, there should be careful planning and readiness. Love and understanding, as well as having positive values towards married life, will result in a happy family that is free from AIDS.

OBJECTIVES:

To be able to:

- *explain why love and understanding will lead to a happy family life.*
- *conduct one's self properly as a good member of the family.*
- *identify what kind of behaviour could lead to an AIDS infection and the destruction of one's family.*
- *develop positive values towards married life, according to Thai customs and culture.*

Teaching activities:

1. Divide the students into five groups.

2. Give a piece of paper to each student to cut according to given patterns 1, 2, and 3.

3. Each group conducts a discussion related to the following topics:

   - *How the first picture is important to the family institution*

   - *How the second picture can be compared to the foundation of society*

   - *How the third picture can be compared to human society*

4. Help students reach the following conclusions:

   - *The first picture demonstrates that a family consists of family members who live happily together.*

   - *The second picture shows that a man and a woman living together to start a family is the foundation of society.*

   - *The third picture shows that people need to live in a social system that encourages good relationships between individuals, and between individuals and different groups in the society.*

5. Distribute worksheets to each group.

6. Group representafives report on the discussion of their respective groups.

- Group 1: How important is it to be ready befoe starting a family.

- Group 2: How do expressions a love and understanding and empathy lead to a happy family life?

- Group 3: How should different family members conduct themselves to bring about family happiness?

  - Father...

  - Mother...

  - Children.......................................

Group 4: How can questionable behaviour by any of the family members risk transmission of AIDS from outside the family?

  - Father...

  - Mother...

  - Children.......................................

- Group 5: Can love, understanding and empathy among family members save one from AIDS? Why?

7. Help the students reach the following conclusions:

For a family to be happy, it should have love and understanding. One should be prepared before starting a family. When there is a problem, people need to discuss it and try to understand one another. In marriage, one needs to have certain positive sexual values and to refrain from sexual promiscuity.

Family members should have mutual empathy, caring, and understanding, and treat one another properly according to their respective roles in the family.

Avoid risky behaviour such as visiting prostitutes, sharing needles for drug use, excessive alcohol consumption, and so on. All these activities can lead to AIDS infection, which can be transmitted to one's spouse, and from a pregnant mother to her foetus.

Adopt the value of monogramy and being faithful to one's spouse. If family problems and sexual problems occur, consult experts or professionals such as doctors, tambon health officers, etc.

Teaching materials:

1. Paper
2. Scissors
3. Worksheet: Samart's problems
4. Self-evaluation form

Evaluation:

1. Observe students' participation, cooperation and enthusiasm in group activities.

2. Check self-evaluation forms.

Suggested additional activities:

1. Summarize ideas into phrases such as share needles, share sex, share AIDS.

2. Write an essay to demonstrate that loving and caring for the home environment can help prevent AIDS.

ACTIVITIES

Paper Cutting

Materials:

1. Three pieces of paper for each student

2. Scissors

Procedure:

Pattern 1

1. Cut the first piece of paper into two parts.

2. Fold the two pieces over and cut following the pattern provided.

Pattern 2

1. Use the second piece of paper. Fold it in half and then into quarters

2. Trace the pictures of a man and a woman on top of the left and right folds as shown below:

3. Cut the paper along the broken line. The result will be two connected figures.

Pattern 3

1. Fold the paper into 8 folds. It should look like an accordion.

2. Trace a male and a female figure on the outermost folds of each end.

3. Fold the paper in one fold at a time and cut along the broken line. When finished, you will have two male figures and two female figures connected to another on each side.

ACTIVITIES

WORKSHEET

Samart's Problems

Directions:

1. Select a group leader and a group secretary.
2. Study "Samart's Problems".
3. Group leader leads the group discussion around these topics:

Group 1 - How important are preparation and readiness before marriage? In which area should one be prepared?

Group 2 - How do expressions of love, understanding and empathy among family members lead to family happiness?

Group 3 - How should one conduct one's self according to his/her place in the family so as to bring about family happiness?

Group 4 - What types of behaviour are risky to contracting AIDS virus and AIDS?

Group 5 - How do love, caring, empathy and understanding within the family help protect a person from AIDS?

4. Each group sends a representative to report to the class.

ACTIVITIES

CASE STUDY: SAMART'S PROBLEMS

Dear Doctor:

I have been following your column for a long time. I have a problem that you might be able to help me with. I am a businessman. I have to travel to the provinces a lot. I stay at home about two days a week. I earn a good income from my business, but my wife doesn't understand me. She thinks I have lovers in the provinces, even though I have always been faithful to her. We frequently argue. I have two teenage children and they are pretty unhappy about it. I am very unhappy and I don't feel like doing my business. Please give me some suggestions so that I can improve my family situation.

Sincerely,

Samart

Dear Khun Samart:

Your problems indicate that you and your wife do not understand each other. I don't know how much love and understanding you and your wife had before marriage and whether there was any planning and preparation for married life, such as knowing each other's habits, building trust, and discussing about sharing your lives. Economic readiness is also an important foundation in marriage. I would like to give you the following advice:

1. You and your wife should face each other and use reason in working out this problem.

2. Give your wife and your children warmth, and regular and sincere demonstrations of your love and understanding.

3. You should know and understand your wife's sexual nature and try to understand each other. If you have any problem, consult your physician.

4. Set a good example for your children by being a good husband. Try to help your wife to understand the nature of your work. Keep her informed of what you are doing to prevent her from being suspicious. Hold to the principle of monogamy and don't be sexually promiscuous. If you cannot avoid sexual encounters outside of marriage, always protect yourself from sexually transmitted diseases which can be passed to your wife especially AIDS, the fatal disease that is spreading right now.

5. You should spend time with your wife and children to develop bonds of love and understanding in order to live happily together.

6. If you set a good example, it will help you teach your children to avoid undesirable behaviours which are prevalent among teenagers. You should be able to be a good advisor to all family members.

7. At present, with AIDS spreading so rapidly, you should give your children advice on ways of protecting themselves from AIDS, such as avoiding sexual promiscuity, not using drugs, and no premarital sex.

I hope this advice is sufficient for now. It you have any more problems, please write to me again. Best wishes to you and your family

Doctor

18

HEALTHY PRACTICES CAN PREVENT AIDS

CONTENT:

Keeping personal items for exclusive use, not sharing or mixing them with those of others is considered good etiquette, and makes good sense. It can protect you from AIDS and other infectious diseases.

OBJECTIVES:

To be able to:

- *identify the value of not sharing one's personal items with others.*
- *identify the dangers of sharing personal items with others.*
- *learn to avoid sharing personal items with others.*

Teaching activities:

Activity 1: Creating a situation

1. Have students from other classes come over to borrow some

personal items while the teacher is teaching, such as shoes, sports uniforms, glasses, erasers, rulers, pens, etc.

2. Engage the class in a discussion about:

   Personal items that can be shared without risk of contracting HIV/AIDS and personal items that should not be shared at all.

3. Present pictures or role play about sharing personal items, for example, people brushing their teeth, a man shaving, a beautician piercing the ears of two children, people sharing a towel, a school girl borrowing a comb from a friend.

   Students should be able to determine which items are personal, and which, if shared, can lead to AIDS infection, and why. Certain personal items may not cause AIDS infection, but may cause other infections. Students should also learn how to politely refuse others from sharing their personal items.

Activity 2: Group Activity

1. Divide the students into three groups to work on three different situations.

Situation 1: Find a nice way to say no to people who ask to share personal items that should not be shared.

Situation 2: The students must be able to determine which personal items can be shared and which cannot.

Situation 3: Make a decision when there is a need to share other people's personal items.

2. Each group sends a group representative to report to the class.

Activity 3: Reaching Conclusions

1. Help the students draw conclusions from Activities 1 and 2. Although being helpful shows generosity, refusing to share

personal items with others is a sound approach to prevent infection from AIDS and other infectious diseases.

2. Have students compile a list of personal items needed at school.

3. Discuss personal items, and identify what students should do at home and at school regarding their use.

4. Have students write down the conclusion.

Activity 4: Homework Assignment

Students are assigned to record their behaviour on the form provided by the teacher.

Teaching materials:

1. Information sheet
2. Worksheets
3. Situations
4. Pictures
5. Self-analysis form

Evaluation:

1. Observation

2. Interview

3. Students' work

4. Behaviour list

ACTIVITIES

Addendum

Prepare instructions and materials for group activities. The worksheets should consist of instruction cards, worksheets, and situations.

Instruction cards:

1. Select group leader and group secretary.
2. Discuss the given situation.
3. Answer the questions.
4. Hand in group work.

Worksheet 1

Members of group 1

1. .... group leader

2. .... group secretary

3. ....

4. ....

5. ....

When you cannot share certain personal items, how should you should say "no"?

1. ....

2. ....

3. ....

4. ....

etc.

Worksheet 2

Members of group 2

1. .... group leader

2. .... group secretary

3. ....

4. ....

5. ....

1. Which personal items can be shared?

   1. ....
   2. ....
   3. ....
   4. ....
   5. ....

2. Which personal items shouldn't be shared with others?

   1. ....
   2. ....
   3. ....
   4. ....
   5. ....

Worksheet 3

Members of Group 3

1. .... group leader

2. .... group secretary

3. ....

4. ....

5. ....

In the event that you can't avoid sharing your personal items with others, what should you do?

....

....

....

....

....

....

ACTIVITIES

Self-Analysis Form

Name .... Number .... Grade 6/ ....

Self Friends Teacher

Behaviour ....

\# 1 # 2 # 3

....

yes no yes no yes no

....

1. Often argue with friends
2. Curse and use bad language
3. Borrow pencils and erasers from classmates
4. Play around during study time
5. Go out at night
6. Ask friends to go out together
7. Steal parents' money
8. Bully friends
9. Take a friend's pen without asking
10. Go out without parent's permission
11. Lie
12. Pick fights with friends
13. Do not do homework
14. Copy homework from friends
15. Refuse to help when on duty
16. Encourage friends to misbehave

19

REASON AND ITS APPLICATION WILL SAVE YOU FROM AIDS

CONTENT:

The ability to think, to make good decisions, to choose what to do, and to live your daily life carefully will protect you from AIDS.

OBJECTIVES:

To be able to:

- *state guidelines for relating with friends from the opposite sex*
- *identify risky behaviour*
- *identify healthy practices that will protect one from AIDS*
- *set a realistic goal for one's family life.*

TEACHING ACTIVITIES:

Activity 1: Group study

1. Divide the students into groups according to sex.

2. Assign worksheets to each group.

3. Present group work to the class.

4. Class discussion and review the dangers and impact of AIDS.

Activity 2: Role playing

1. Create a situation depicting a New Year's celebration. Two young people who are interested in one another often go out alone at night. However, there are different expectations between a boy and a girl. She perceives love as a source of emotional warmth, whereas the boy perceives love as an expression of sexual desire and need. The girl is asked to go to the boy's home. Being close together leads to a sexual relationship that the girl does not plan to have. It is very sad to find out later that the girl is infected with the AIDS virus. She may also be pregnant and may transmit the virus to the foetus.

2. Ask for volunteers to role play or present a skit. The teacher helps the students with the script and direction.

3. Discuss the following topics:

   1. If you had been the girl in the skit, what would you have said to get yourself out of a sexual encounter?

      Possible answers:

      - Ask for sympathy.
      - Tell him you are menstruating.
      - Tell him you have AIDS.
      - Tell him you will call the police for help.

   2. If you were a pregnant girl with AIDS and you were not certain whether the baby would have AIDS, what would you do and how would you feel?

Possible answers

- Anxious and worried, and would go to the doctor.

- Sad and would consult parents.

- Cynically pleased and stay pregnant. etc.

3. Why does this kind of situation happen to a woman? How can it be prevented?

Possible answers:

3.1 The woman should:

- refuse to go with the man alone.
- agree to go but go with other friends.
- agree to go but together with adults.
- agree to go except to isolated places.

3.2 The man should:

- understand the girl's feelings, her being worried and being afraid of getting pregnant and/or becoming infected, or that her parents will find out.

- have a sexual relationship only when he and his partner are ready and know how to protect themselves.

4. What should be one's goal for having a family?

Possible answers:

- Choose a good person to be a spouse.
- Get married only when ready.
- Have blood tests before marriage. etc.

5. Class discussion and summary.

Activity 3: Homework assignment

Write an essay entitled, "When you have a relative who has AIDS".

It should be about one to two pages in length. The essay should include what you should do if you have to live with a person who has AIDS.

Teaching materials:

1. Situations and role playing.
2. Worksheets.

Evaluation:

1. Observe the students' participation in group discussion, presentation, and role playing.
2. Students' answers.
3. Group work
4. Essay.

Suggested additional activities:

1. Use school radio to broadcast AIDS information.
2. Arrange an information corner on how to protect one's self from AIDS.

ACTIVITIES

Worksheet

GROUP 1: *MALE STUDENTS*

1. Select group leader and group secretary.
2. Hold group discussion on given situations.
3. Record summary of group discussion.
4. Hand in group work.

Situation:

AIDS can spread to all strata of society, to people of both sexes and from all walks of life. It may happen accidentally or consciously such as by coming into contact with or receiving transfusion, or through transmission from an AIDS-infected mother to her baby of AIDS-infected blood. If you want to be free from AIDS, what should you do to avoid it?

....

....

....

GROUP 2: *FEMALE STUDENTS*

1. Select group leader and group secretary.
2. Hold group discussion on given situations
3. Record summary of group discussion.
4. Hand in group work.

Situation:

There is a fatal disease called AIDS that is spreading rapidly. It can be transmitted to anybody. Students should learn how it is transmitted and what kind of behaviour puts one at risk for the infection. Risky behaviour includes having indiscriminate sexual relations, premarital sex, being raped and being a prostitute. If you are deceived, how would you solve the problem in a way that would save your life?

....

....

....

....

....

....

20

SELF-CONTROL CAN PREVENT ONE FROM CONTRACTING AIDS

CONTENT:

Practising self-control and mindfulness can help protect a person from being infected with AIDS.

OBJECTIVE:

To be able to:

- *state the meaning and the benefits of being mindful;*
- *give examples of mindful conduct;*
- *know what one should do to avoid contracting AIDS.*

Teaching activities:

1. Play the game Land, Water, and Air.

   Have a student say land, water or air and ask another student to respond by naming an animal that belongs to the category stated (that is, land, water or air), within the count of three. If the student gives a wrong answer or is not able to answer within the time limit, he or she loses. Repeat until every student has a chance to participate. The animal names cannot be repeated.

2. Ask students to state the benefits of playing the game, such as fun, mental training, memory training, training in being mindful, and etc.

3. Relate the definition of mindfulness to its application.

   Mindfulness means being conscious of what you think and what you do. Man's conscience controls human behaviour and brings about success. A mindful person is a person who does things with care, and with self-control so that he always does the right things.

   Name some distinguished persons in the community whom students can use as role models.

4. Divide the students into four groups to work on the worksheet shown in "Activities".

ACTIVITIES

Worksheet

GROUP ....

Mindful behaviour includes:

1. Looking left and right before crossing the street;
2. Seeing a person electrocuted, save him in the most effective manner;
3. ....
4. ....

Careless behaviour includes:

1. Drinking while driving;

2. Feeling so disappointed after failing an exam that you decide not to go back to school;

3. ....

4. ....

5. Have each group study the situation below, then answer the questions.

....

Jirapong, Sophon, Wichien, and Paiboon are close friends studying in grade 6. Sophon is a very good student but he likes to go out for a good time. Paiboon is a moderately good student; he is very weak-willed. Wichien is a poor student but quiet and hard working. Jirapong is reasonable, generous and well-liked.

Two days before the final exam, while Wichien and Jirapong are studying for the exam, Sophon and Paiboon invite them to go to the annual village fair. A famous singer is performing and every one wants to go except Jirapong, who says, "I don't think we should go. We might fail the exam. This is a very important exam." Sophon insists; he says "It shouldn't matter. We have been studying hard all year. Just going out for one night won't make us fail." Wichien gives in to his friends but Jirapong decides to stay home and study.

Discuss the situation covering the following topics:

1. What values does Jirapong base his decision on?

2. What are the benefits of such a decision?

6. From Activity 5, point out the importance of self-control and mindfulness. In addition, students need to develop other values and characteristics, such as wisdom, care, knowing what is right and what is wrong, patience, self-discipline, respecting the laws and rules of society and obedience. AIDS

is a fatal disease for which there is no cure. There are a lot of people infected with the AIDS virus and people who have full blown AIDS. How should students exercise self-control so that they will not be infected?

7. Have students analyze, from Module 8, how men and women view the concept of love, which may be summarized as follows:

    1. One needs to keep up with new information about AIDS and its prevention.
    2. Be a role model for others in the prevention of AIDS.
    3. Cooperate with various agencies working in AIDS prevention.
    4. Do not use drugs.
    5. Do not do anything that can cause infection, such as having casual sexual relations.
    6. Do not share sharp objects that have not been disinfected, such as razors and needles.
    7. Refuse to do things that are improper.
    8. If you think you might have been infected, go to a hospital to have blood tests.
    9. Others

8. Students and teacher agree to do the right thing at home and at school and to try to practice being mindful whenever possible.

9. Record the summary in notebooks.

Teaching materials:

1. Instruction cards

2. Situations and news
3. Diagrams of summary

Evaluation:

1. Observe students' behaviour from the Activity Record Form.
2. Check students' work.

Suggested additional activities:

1. Arrange the bulletin board.
2. Essay contest.
3. Slogan contest.
4. Research for more information.

ACTIVITIES

Activities Record Form

Name .... Grade ....

Record your daily agreed-upon behaviour and actions.

....

Date	Activities at school	Activities at home
....	....	....
....	....	....
....	....	....
....	....	....

21

LEADING AN ETHICAL LIFE HELPS PREVENT AIDS

CONTENT:

To behave righteously means to do things that do not cause trouble and suffering to others. If one has self-control and does the right thing, the result will be a good life, one that is free from AIDS.

Objectives:

To be able to:

- *give examples of values helpful in preventing AIDS.*
- *state the benefit of leading a righteous life (being mindful, responsible, ashamed to do anything wrong)*
- *conduct one's self according to the Dharma in order to be free from AIDS.*

Teaching activities:

1. Review information about AIDS using a video tape or created situation about the feelings of those close to a person who

died of AIDS. Point out feelings of sympathy, and the desire to be helpful and to help prevent AIDS.

2. Divide the students into three groups to discuss Somsri's case according to these given topics:

    - What would you do if you had been Somsri, other than committing suicide?

    - This kind of thing happens because of the lack of certain values. What are they?

    - How can these values be developed?

3. Have students analyze this statement "From a survey, it has been found that people who are HIV positive and people who have AIDS include men and women from different age groups and from different professions."

    From the above statement, we can say that even educated people can be infected if they don't protect themselves.

    Have students discuss the following topics:

    - If you know something is wrong, why do you still do it?

    - How would you correct that kind of conduct?

    - Draw up some guidelines of what you should do and what you are able to do.

    - Have all students agree to follow the guidelines.

    The teacher points out to the students that everybody is different so levels of achievement varies from person to person. However, everyone has to follow the guidelines, guide and help one another to complete the task.

4. Have the students state their responsibility in fighting AIDS.

5. Help the students reach the following conclusion:

Even educated people can be infected with AIDS if they do not apply their learning in their life. We should be sympathetic to people who are infected with the AIDS virus and should take part in AIDS prevention work. We should have correct information about the disease by following development concerning AIDS and protecting ourselves from AIDS by being mindful and refusing to do wrong things.

Teaching materials:

1. Video tape or situation
2. Worksheet
3. News clippings
4. Self-evaluation form

Evaluation:

1. Observe the students' behaviour based on the self-analysis form.
2. Conduct an interview, asking the following questions. Have students write the answers in their notebooks.
    - *What are the values that aré beneficial to the prevention of AIDS?*
    - *What behaviour is useful in preventing AIDS?*
    - *What are your responsibilities in the prevention of AIDS?*

Student's answers may include the following:

1. Learn as much as possible about AIDS.
2. Follow the news about AIDS.

3. Inform people you know about AIDS, its transmission and prevention whenever there is an opportunity.

4. Be helpful and supportive to people who have AIDS.

5. Protect yourself from AIDS.

6. Try to protect people close to you or people who exhibit risky behaviour by giving advice and by encouraging them to do the right thing and to eliminate or reduce undesirable behaviour]

Suggested Additional Activities:

1. Have the students search for more information from different sources and present it to the class.

2. Divide the students into groups and have them organize an exhibition.

3. Invite a resource person to give a lecture.

ACTIVITIES

WORKSHEET

Case study

Somsri came from a poor family. After school, she had to sell flowers to support her family. Her mother was sick and she had several younger siblings. Her father left the family for another woman and never sent them money. One day, while on her way home, she was accosted and nearly raped but she was saved in time.

She felt vew dicouraged and hopeless, as though she were a bad person. She didn't understand why something like that happened to her since she had never caused trouble to anybody. She had always suffered for the sake of her family. She felt so bad about herself that she tried to commit suicide, but somebody saved her again.

Discuss the following topics:

1. *If you were Somsri, what would you do with your life instead of trying to commit suicide?*

2. *This happened because people lacked certain ethical values. What are they?*

3. *How can those values be developed?*

Report your answers to the class for further discussion.

ACTIVITIES

Self-analysis form

Name .... Grade ....

Explain why certain kinds of behaviour are beneficial and why certain behaviours need improvement. Use the list below:

....

Behaviour	Benefit	Need improvement
....	....	....
....	....	....
Personal		
....	....	....
....	....	....
....	....	....
Towards others		
....	....	....
....	....	....
....	....	....

Signature ....

Date ....

ACTIVITIES

Self-evaluation form

Name .... Grade ....

Make an × in front of the statements that are consistent with your characteristics.

.... Responsible

.... Am a trusting person

.... Reasonable

.... Make acquaintances easily

.... Do not like to work

.... Like to be in fashion

.... Like to be helped

.... Like to help others

.... Like to go out

.... Like nature

.... Like to walk in shopping stalls

.... Get angry easily

.... Easily bothered

.... Impatient

.... Like to take action instead of talking

.... Like to do housework

.... Like to imitate movie stars

Signature ....

Date ....